This book is dedicated to all cancer patients and their caregivers who demonstrate the strength to fight cancer every day.

THE STRENGTH TO FIGHT CANCER
A FAMILY GUIDE

A publication of the Quality of Life Foundation
115 West 19th Street
Indianapolis, IN 46202
317-924-4022

Authors
Dale E. Theobald, Ph.D., M.D.,
William M. Dugan, Jr., M.D.,
Judy Burnett,
Abby A. Marmion,
and Sara Edgerton, M.S.

Printed by Ripon Community Printers
656 South Douglas St., P.O. Box 6
Ripon, WI
Printed in the United States of America
Second Printing, May, 2003

ISBN 0-9720935-1-6

CONTENTS

FORWARD

Jill Eikenberry & Michael Tucker

We discovered The Quality of Life Foundation a little over three years ago — or perhaps they discovered us, I'm not sure. But it was love at first sight. Their humane and holistic attitude toward the event of cancer — their regard for the emotional and spiritual well-being of the patient as well as that of the patient's family and friends — is something we fully support. When we went through our experience with cancer, attitudes towards complementary care were in the dark ages. We felt alone, terrified, bullied by physicians who meant well but had no regard for what we were going through emotionally.

When Jill was about to go into the operating room, the doctor told me to wait downstairs and that they would meet me there in about two hours. I waited eight and one-half hours — no one would give me any information — the most dire scenarios paraded through my brain as the clock slowly ticked by. When they finally came down, I rushed to the doctor in a panic and asked him what had happened. "Oh, we had a traffic jam," he said casually. "We didn't go in until a couple of hours ago."

Jill had a similar experience two days later as she tensely awaited the results of her node involvement. The doctor came into her room to check her sutures — Jill knew he must have the results of the nodes — and he said nothing. Finally, as he was leaving, she got up the courage to ask him and as an afterthought, he tossed off, "Oh, you're fine."

Cancer is scary — not just for the person receiving the diagnosis, but for all the people who love her and, in the case of spouses and children, depend on her to be around.

"The Strength to Fight Cancer" is a virtual roadmap to the understanding of the cancer experience. It approaches cancer on human terms. It is invaluable to anyone who has received a diagnosis of cancer and a lifeline for those loved ones who are trying to help, trying to understand, and trying to cope.

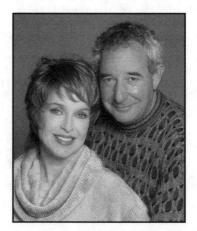

PREFACE
THE STRENGTH TO FIGHT CANCER
A FAMILY GUIDE

Whether it's through a personal experience, or the experience of a family member or friend, many people are touched in some way by cancer. There are one million new cancer cases diagnosed every year in the United States. There are over 11 million cancer survivors living in the U.S. today. Because of early detection and more effective treatment therapies, cancer today has, in many cases, been transformed from an *acute life-threatening illness to a chronic* (and many times life-threatening) *illness.*

For patients with many types of cancer, survival rates today are much better. Cancer patients are living longer. Cancer is now thought of as a "treatable" illness, rather than a disease that may or may not be "curable."

With this increase in survival, the importance of symptom control and supportive therapies to maintain quality of life for patients has increased. In the last ten years, great strides have been made in the development of strategies that can be used to control these symptoms, and thus, improve the quality of life for the patient. Efforts that focus on enabling patients to participate in activities of daily living are of key importance.

This book is written for those whose lives are touched by cancer: cancer survivors, patients, family members, caregivers, friends, and loved ones. Cancer affects these people in many different ways. While there are hundreds of books available about cancer, the authors felt a need existed for a simple guide (in simple terms) to help people understand how to take an active role in cancer care and treatment. Whether it's for the patient himself, or a loved one as the caregiver, this guide will help to navigate the uncertain waters of cancer. Knowledge empowers patients and families.

Each author has been touched by cancer in a different way. Whether as a member of an oncology care team or as a family member of someone who has had cancer, each person has provided a unique and personal perspective.

We dedicate this book to all cancer patients, their caregivers, and their loved ones who demonstrate the strength to fight cancer every day.

Special thanks to
Randall Trowbridge, M.D.
and Roberta Szumski, R.N.
for reviewing this manuscript.

CHAPTER 1
WHEN YOUR DOCTOR SAYS IT'S CANCER

When the doctor says "you have cancer" it is not unusual for patients to experience intense emotional and even physical reactions. Cancer can change everything in our lives. It can change our life plans. It can threaten previously stable financial plans. It can even challenge our faith. Dr. Jimmie C. Holland has written about some of these fears. She calls them the "5D's" and sees them as the most common fears cancer patients have. Let's review them now.

What are the 5D's?
Death
Does having this illness mean that I am going to die? How will I die?

Dependence
Will I have to be dependent upon my friends and
      family members?
Will I be a burden to others?
Will I lose my independence?

Disruption
Will my life be disrupted?
Will I disrupt the lives of others?

Disability
Will I be able to go to work?
Will I have enough money?
Will I be able to carry on with my daily activities?
Will my illness physically disable me and will
      people notice?

Disfigurement
Will I look different?
Will my co-workers and friends notice that something
      is wrong with me?
Will my spouse or partner reject me?

These are all real concerns and very common questions that patients with a serious illness often ask themselves.

The 5D's and Symptoms
Dealing with the 5D's of illness can become stressful and often overwhelming for patients. This may lead to emotional issues such as fear, anxiety, and depression. As a family member and caregiver, just understanding what the patient may be experiencing is the first step to helping them cope with the challenges.

How Do I Help?

Cancer is not contagious. It is important to be "present" for the patient. That is a fancy way of telling you to be available physically and emotionally. Be a good listener. If the news from the doctor is bad, don't be afraid to listen and just be there for the patient. There are probably no magical or profound words to say. It's okay for your loved one to "not like it." That is a common reaction. Communicating by your presence and lack of avoidance is most important.

Timing is also key. Even the most well adjusted people need time to accept bad news about their health. Early on, they may not want to talk about it. Later, however, they may want to talk about it over and over. Let them set the pace. We all need consistent, loving support. One of your roles as a caregiver should be to help the patient plan for the worst, hope for the best.

CHAPTER 2
TALKING TO YOUR DOCTORS AND YOUR NURSES

When a patient is presented with the news of a serious illness, they often feel that their world has been turned upside down. It is very important for family members and significant others to get involved and ensure that the patient's needs and concerns are properly communicated to the healthcare team. How well you, the patient, and the health care team talk to each other is one of the most important parts of getting good medical care. This will take some pre-planning and effort on your part to accomplish this, but it is time well spent.

Doing Your Homework
Understanding the treatment process and making sure the physicians and nurses understand the patient's needs are important factors in getting successful medical treatment for any illness. Think of it as forming a partnership with them and working together to solve problems. In today's world, physicians' visits with patients are typically brief. This is an incredibly

small amount of time compared to years ago when doctors used to make house calls. Many times, a routine office visit may last only 15 minutes. And, this does not necessarily mean 15 minutes of time with the doctor. Other things must occur during this visit, such as talking to the nurse, taking the patient's vital signs, and other activities that are necessary for patient care.

This time constraint is driven by factors such as medical insurance reimbursement and is often outside the doctor's control. Therefore, you will need to get the most from the time you and the patient spend with the doctor by doing some "homework" before the appointments. Doing this homework will help to further educate both of you. Typically, the more educated a patient is about the illness, the better the care he gets.

Taking an Active Role
Part of doing your homework can be to take an active role in the patient's care and treatment by acting as a second pair of eyes and ears, which will enable him to focus on his treatment. Become an "expert" on the cancer – learn as much as you can about the patient's illness. Gather information from your local health care team, the American Cancer Society and other support groups in your area. If you have access to the Internet, use this cautiously as an additional resource. There are many websites that provide good patient

information — and there are just as many that give bad advice. Chapter 14 of this guide provides a listing of websites that are good resources.

One of the most important factors in getting good medical care is preparing for doctor appointments. Before seeing a specialist, be sure to buy a journal or notebook to be used specifically for the patient's doctor visits so you can take notes for the patient. You may also use the note pages at the back of this book. This allows the patient to listen to the physician without worrying about writing anything down. Keeping one journal/notebook with entries in chronological order will enable you to follow the treatment process more easily and refer back to conversations with the health care team. Be sure to list the day, date, and year of each appointment in the journal.

Prior to doctor appointments, write any questions or concerns you or the patient may have in the journal so that you are prepared before seeing the doctor. Read any printed literature you may have collected about the cancer, and bring this with you to the appointment in order to have a productive conversation with the doctor and nurse. Again, write down any questions you may have about this literature.

Getting Started With a New Doctor

The first meeting with a new doctor is the best time to begin communicating openly and positively. An important thing to remember is to not be intimidated by the medical treatment process. Doctors possess a wealth of knowledge, so think of them as a resource for you and the patient. Ask the doctor if it is ok to audio tape him during the first meeting. This may be helpful to review later. Be sure to introduce yourself and tell the doctor your relationship to the patient – and the role you will be taking in his treatment. Get to know the names of the nurses and others on the health care team so they recognize you and the patient when you come in the next time.

Understanding the patient's treatment goals and values is an important component of communication. You should also understand the doctor's treatment goals and values to facilitate a good working relationship. Depending upon the type of cancer and the stage of the illness, patients may have different goals and thoughts about their treatment. Some may want to do anything possible to reduce the cancer, while others in a more advanced stage may be more concerned with maintaining the best quality-of-life possible. Discussing these goals and values together with the patient and the doctors/nurses will help to get everyone on the same page and open the lines of communication.

This may be an appropriate time to discuss the prognosis — or expected outcome of the cancer — with your health care team. Ask your doctors and nurses about the specific expectations about the illness and the treatment. There are many misconceptions in the general public regarding the prognosis of cancer. Cancer is not a disease – rather it is made up of more than 100 diseases with thousands of variations, each of which require its own individual treatment approach. Some cancers develop extremely slowly, while others are much more aggressive in nature.

Often times, the perception is that a patient with an advanced stage of cancer is going to die, when in reality, this may not be true at all.

For both you and the patient, knowing what to expect at the beginning of an illness can make it easier to cope and prepare. Again, preparing questions you and the patient may have ahead of time will maximize your time with the doctors.

The Doctor Works For You
At times, you and the patient may feel bashful about taking the doctor's time in order to ask questions or talk through issues about the illness. Just remember one thing: you are paying the doctor for his expertise and services. Be assertive, and get satisfactory answers

before leaving the doctor's office. Don't treat this any differently than you would if you were hiring another type of expert to perform a job or a service.

If the doctor absolutely cannot spend the time needed with you and the patient, ask to speak to the nurse or nurse practitioner, or schedule a family conference with the doctor.

Getting Second Opinions

Having confidence in the type of care the patient is receiving is very important. Many times, patients and families need clarification and want to know that everything possible is being done to get the best, most appropriate cancer care.

If you or the patient is not completely satisfied with the doctor, the diagnosis/prognosis, or treatment recommendations, or just want a confirmation of the information, it may be an appropriate time to consider getting another opinion from a second doctor.

While this may initially put you in an uncomfortable situation with the current doctor, it will give you and the patient the peace of mind you need to move ahead in the care process. Have a discussion with your family doctor about your concerns, and ask for further recommendations and names of other specialists.

A good rule of thumb is that any doctor who does not support a caregiver or patient seeking a second opinion may not be worth a first opinion.

Caregiver Tips
- If you have questions about specific tests or treatment, be sure to ask. That way, you have an idea before you leave.

- Ask for a copy of the patient's test results throughout the treatment process. Ask your doctor to explain what these results mean in the context of the overall treatment. Be sure to make notes in the patient's journal/notebook.

- Attend as many of the doctor visits or treatment sessions as you can. You can act as a second set of ears for the patient.

- Throughout the course of treatment, tell your doctor/nurse team about any side effects the patient is having. Many times, patients have the expectation that because they are ill, they should automatically experience pain, fatigue, depression, or other side effects. These are all treatable – but the doctor needs to know about side effects in order to help the patient.

- Get to know the nurse team, and encourage the patient to do the same. During the cancer treatment process, the patient will spend the majority of his time with the oncology nursing staff – especially if he is going to have chemotherapy. The nurses can be a wonderful support mechanism and resource.

- During the course of the treatment process, let the doctor know how things are going and how it is affecting the patient's family members.

- Talk to other people in your community with similar illnesses. You will be surprised by the information you can glean from them, however, understand cancer affects everyone in different ways.

- Try not to hover over the patient. He will still need to feel he has independence and decision-making capabilities.

- Let the doctor know who has Power of Attorney for the patient or who will officially serve as the Health Care Representative.

A FAMILY MEMBER'S PERSPECTIVE

Kris, whose mother had lung cancer, had different communication experiences with different doctors.

"When my mother's surgeon came in to tell us that her tumor was malignant and not removable, he sure lacked any bedside manner. I remember he kept backing out the doorway of her hospital room all the time he was talking. It was as if he was running away from answering the tough questions.

"Then, the medical oncologist scheduled a meeting with my sister, brother, and me. Wow, what a difference! He started the meeting by asking us to tell him about our mom. He spent an hour with us, learning about her, about her wishes and about our wishes. It was a completely different experience and one I felt really good about. I felt like he cared about my mom, even though he had just met her for the first time. He had one of the hospital social workers attend that meeting with us. It was great because she became a source of information and support during the month in the hospital. Just having her help coordinate moving my mom home was a big relief. And, I always knew I could call the oncologist any time I had a question. He was great.

"I would tell anyone to make sure you have physicians involved in your case that you feel like you can talk to. It is so important to be able to ask whatever questions you may have. The answers don't always have to come from the doctor. A nurse or a social worker can be very helpful and usually have more time to spend with you."

CHAPTER 3
THE EMOTIONAL CHALLENGES

In recent years, there has been an increased focus on symptom management in cancer patients. Patients in general are living longer than they were years ago. Also, there is now increased focus on symptom management and quality-of-life. It is very important to begin symptom management early in the treatment process. If left untreated, these symptoms can significantly impair a patient's quality-of-life and cause him to function at a lower level in daily activities.

Cancer is an illness that causes many symptoms. In addition to the physical symptoms that cancer and its treatment can cause, emotional symptoms occur in many patients as well. Providing comfort, relieving symptoms, and easing distress caused from cancer and its treatment is known as symptom management. This type of care is important during *all* stages of cancer treatment and is aimed at controlling symptoms and improving quality-of-life. It also addresses the family's needs throughout the course of the illness.

Participating in symptom management is of key importance because it enables the patient to focus his time on feeling better.

Two of the most common emotional symptoms of cancer are *anxiety* and *depression*. These symptoms change over time. When patients learn they have cancer, they can react intensely with anger, panic, fear, and denial. These reactions can lead to even more extreme behaviors such as avoiding people, sleeping, and intense episodes of crying. For some patients, these intense reactions can occur after an initial diagnosis of cancer or after learning of a recurrence of the illness. After this, patients typically enter an adaptive phase and become more centered on their treatment and learning about the illness.

Anxiety

Anxiety is a normal reaction to cancer. It is an emotional reaction to fear and causes the body to respond as though it were under physical attack. This symptom may occur after a diagnosis, while awaiting test results, while undergoing treatment, or from anticipating a recurrence of the illness. Anxiety may cause the heart to beat faster, a rise in blood pressure, stress hormones (such as adrenaline) to be released into the system and may make the palms sweat. It can also cause worry and panic, interfere with sleep, cause nausea and vomiting, and severely decrease a patient's quality-of-life and ability to function properly.

Patients may experience fear, be unable to absorb and understand information they receive from their health care team, or even be unable to go through with treatment. Anxiety levels differ in each individual patient, and most patients are able to reduce their level of anxiety by learning more about their cancer, the treatment, and the doctor's prognosis. For some patients who have experienced intense anxiety prior to cancer diagnosis, feelings of anxiety may become more intense. Patients who have not had episodes of anxiety during other parts of their life will typically deal better with anxiety related to their cancer. Intense anxiety is more likely to occur in patients who have a history of anxiety episodes or are experiencing anxiety when they are initially diagnosed with cancer.

These symptoms are common side effects of having a life-threatening illness as well as going through cancer treatment. Anxiety can be treated in different ways. Medications, quality-of-life counseling, hypnosis, or a combination of these methods are commonly used.

Mood swings can be expected when coping with a life-threatening illness, but if feelings of anxiety last longer than two or three weeks, begin to increase in intensity, or prevent patients from participating in normal daily activities, you should talk to your health care team about depression. During an illness, anxiety can lead to depressive symptoms and depression.

Higher Anxiety Time Periods

Anxiety levels can become especially high for patients during the time periods between tests. This is one element they worry about most. They worry about things like whether the cancer will recur, or whether the treatment is effective, or what happens if the treatment is unsuccessful. It is important that you understand the patient may need to share their anxieties about this with you. The best thing you can do as a caregiver is listen.

Depression

Depression is a common side effect of cancer and its treatment. Studies show that 50% of cancer patients show mild to moderate symptoms of anxiety and depressive behavior. About 20% - 25% have more severe depression. Depression can have very negative effects on quality-of-life and significantly impair a patient's ability to continue working, participate with family, make health care decisions, and have social relationships. Depression may be effectively treated. It's important that it be discussed early on.

If a patient has been depressed in the past or has a family history of depression, he is more likely to become depressed as he works through his experience with cancer.

Depression is difficult to diagnose because it can be confused with feeling bad and other problems associated with cancer and its treatment. The side effects of treatment can often look like depression. Fatigue, for example, a direct side effect of cancer treatment, can be mistaken for depression. Fatigue may cause a person to feel tired, weak, exhausted, weary, worn-out, fatigued, heavy, or slow — all symptoms that a depressed patient may experience. Fatigue will be covered in more detail in the next chapter, "The Physical Challenges".

If the patient feels sad and low most of the time, it is possible he has become depressed. Depression isn't a sign of personal failure or inability to cope, rather it is an illness, and it can often be triggered by the emotional stresses of cancer and its treatment. Some of the key symptoms of depression include experiencing a low mood for long periods of time, not feeling like your usual self, inability to boost out of a low mood, lack of enjoyment in and losing interest in your favorite activities. These symptoms are often accompanied by other symptoms, such as anxiety, hopelessness, guilt, sleeplessness, inability to concentrate, fatigue, lack of motivation, loss of self-esteem, and thoughts of death or suicide.

Depression affects daily living and the ability to function. It can also destroy quality-of-life if left untreated. If a patient has been depressed in the past or has a family history of depression, the risk for developing depressive symptoms is greater. There are a number of treatments for depression that can dramatically improve quality-of-life. Patients may need to see a mental health professional such as a psychiatrist or psychologist – preferably one who has experience with physical and life-threatening illnesses. Anti-depressants may be recommended and are generally very effective, tolerated well by patients, and are not drugs of abuse. Depression can also be managed through psychotherapy, other medication, support groups, or a combination of these efforts. Many people feel embarrassed to admit they feel depressed, but seeking help is important and becoming commonplace.

Be sure to encourage the patient to talk to the doctors and nurses if he is experiencing depressive symptoms. They can help only if they know how the patient is feeling.

A PATIENT'S PERSPECTIVE

Pat discovered she had breast cancer eight months after having a quadruple bypass. Then, several months later, her husband was diagnosed with prostate cancer. At the same time she was dealing with an aging parent.

"I was totally surprised. I had just had a quadruple bypass about eight months before and then I went in for a routine mammogram. The doctor's office called and said it had to be repeated – that something looked different. I really wasn't worried about it at this point. I had another mammogram, an ultrasound and a needle biopsy. When the doctor called and said it was definitely cancer I was stunned. Fortunately it had not spread. I was given three choices: have radiation and take a drug called Tamoxifen for 5 years, have a mastectomy and take Tamoxifen for five years, or have both breasts removed and not have to take Tamoxifen. I chose the double mastectomy and I did not want to have reconstructive surgery – I'd had enough surgery.

"A few months ago I started seeing a psychiatrist for depression. I felt I couldn't get anything done. I wasn't getting any sleep. I kept thinking it was going to get better. I didn't think I was depressed but my daughter and my surgeon thought I should see someone. After a few sessions with the psychiatrist I realized I really was

depressed. The sessions with the psychiatrist are helping. I was taking an anti-depressant for awhile and that really helped but I had some side effects. My psychiatrist is going to put me on something else. As I think back, I think my depression started with the bypass surgery. Then, with my husband's cancer and my elderly mother's health problems, I was worried about who was going to take care of everyone if I couldn't. I just felt overwhelmed by the responsibility. It has been unbelievably helpful to work through all this with the psychiatrist."

CHAPTER 4
THE PHYSICAL CHALLENGES

In addition to the emotional challenges of cancer and its treatment, there are also physical challenges. Many cancer treatments may include surgery to remove a tumor, chemotherapy, or radiation. Seventy to 85% of all people with cancer receive some combination of treatments, either as the primary therapy or the therapy for a recurrent tumor. Many times, these treatments have uncomfortable side effects. The cancer itself can also cause side effects. Some of the most common are pain, fatigue, nausea, vomiting, loss-of-appetite, and "chemo fuzzies". Many times these are temporary and can be alleviated with medication or other types of therapies.

Pain
Pain management has become a higher priority in our country during the last several years, and, health care policymakers, health care professionals, regulators, and the general public have increasingly taken an interest in providing better pain therapies. In 1999, the

Joint Commission of Accreditation of Healthcare Organizations developed new standards that created new expectations for assessing and managing pain in both the hospital and other health care settings. The new standards acknowledged that pain accompanies a number of diseases and injuries including cancer, and requires explicit attention.

One of the first things people with advanced cancer worry about is pain. Approximately 60% of patients with advanced stages of cancer experience pain, however, there are medications to control this side effect. To ensure an active role in decision making, patients should consider allowing a family member or close friend to learn as much as possible about pain treatment.

Whatever strategy is used to treat pain, the doctors, nurses, and caregivers must work together. Oncologists must work hand-in-hand with nurses, primary care physicians, and other caregivers on the health care team such as psychologists or therapists to provide *consistent* and *aggressive* pain relief. If treatment is fragmented, the patient may suffer simply due to inconsistency.

Proper pain management is very important. The following "4As" of pain management, developed by two authors who have written about cancer pain, can be used by doctors as a guide to determine the effectiveness of a cancer patient's pain program.

Analgesia: is the patient getting pain relief?

Activities of Daily Living: can the patient function properly each day?

Adverse events: is the patient having side effects from the pain medication?

Aberrant behavior: is the patient misusing or mis-taking the pain medicine due to inadequate pain control?

Measuring these outcomes is an important part of determining the success of a patient's overall pain management program and should be discussed on a regular basis with the doctor.

"I Don't Want to Be Addicted to Drugs"

Cancer can cause pain. Many times patients do not want to take pain medicine because they will become "addicted", and sometimes caregivers withhold pain medicine for the same reason — they do not want the patient to become "addicted". Unfortunately these fears can lead to enormous unnecessary suffering and loss of quality-of-life. Untreated pain causes people to withdraw from life's sustaining activities, both social and vocational. Over time, untreated pain doubles the risk of depression, further impairing the patient's ability to function. Withholding of pain medication including strong opioid (narcotic) medication comes from a lack of understanding of terms and unfounded fears. There are three terms that must be understood when considering uses of pain medication: dependence, addiction, and tolerance. We will discuss them here.

Dependence. Every patient that takes opioid based medication for a significant period of time will become dependent upon the medication. That is a natural consequence of taking the medicine. It simply means that if the patient stops taking the medication suddenly, he will have withdrawal symptoms. These symptoms may be mild, or they may be very uncomfortable and dangerous. When these medicines are stopped, they must be tapered. Tapering is not dangerous and is commonly done in pain management. In this case, the patient is taking medication under the supervision of a doctor for a medical reason.

Addiction. Addiction has a very different meaning. Addiction is the use of medication for *non-medical* reasons such as selling the medicine for money, trading the medicine for other medicine, giving the medicine to friends, taking the medicine for reasons other than pain (sleeplessness or avoidance of stress), or having drug parties. The likelihood of someone doing these things who does not already have a history of addiction is extremely low — nearly non-existent. It is certainly not enough of a risk that a patient should suffer with severe pain. Sometimes patients who have strong history of addiction get cancer and need pain medication. These patients can be treated safely but they require extra attention, and they must be treated for the addiction. Sometimes patients who are not following doctor's orders by taking too much medicine or demanding more medicine are not addicted — their pain is simply under treated and they need to be re-evaluated. This is a difficult judgment and must be made by the doctor.

Tolerance. When a new medication is started, the patient's body is not used to it. A small amount of medication may work. As one's system "gets use to" the medicine, the dose may need to be increased to have the same effect. This is a natural process that occurs in our bodies. It does not mean that the patient is asking for more medication to get even a stronger effect. It means that more medication may be needed to have the same effect. This process will not continue on and on. Eventually a stable dose will be achieved.

Confusion about these three terms frequently leads to poor pain control — a very unfortunate result for the patient. Finally, pain medication has side effects such as sedation, constipation, fatigue, and sometimes confusion. It is important to be aware of these and plan for them. Pain management should be a regular topic at the doctor's visits if pain is a problem. Other interventions may be useful to manage pain. Massage, relaxation, imagery, and hypnosis are examples of other treatments that may be useful. When they fail, pain medication should not be withheld.

When cancer pain changes in intensity, location, or duration, the automatic response should not be to increase the medication. There are other interventions such as radiation therapy, chemotherapy, and even surgery that may be helpful or required. Pain management is an active process with ongoing monitoring by the patient's medical team.

Fatigue

Tiredness, or fatigue, during chemotherapy treatment is common and can be overwhelming if not diagnosed and treated. Fatigue is the most common symptom associated with cancer and its treatment — affecting about 90% of all cancer patients at some time during their illness. Fatigue can be described as an excessive overall body tiredness or weariness that is not relieved by sleep or rest. Fatigue may be short or long-term, depending on the type of treatments patients are undergoing. Fatigue affects everyone in different ways.

Some patients find they have very mild fatigue, and it does not interfere with their daily activities. For others, fatigue can be very disruptive. If left untreated, it can have a negative impact on quality-of-life and can affect the patient's family members as well.

There are many ways to handle fatigue. The first and most important step is narrowing down the cause of fatigue. It can result from various sources such as surgery, chemotherapy, radiation, hormonal therapies, anemia, or excessive medications. Fatigue caused by some of these treatments can be treated by specific medications. It is important to discuss this with your medical team. Besides medical interventions, there are some environmental/lifestyle changes that may help.

Managing the Effects of Fatigue
Planning ahead both at home and at work is important in managing fatigue. Help the patient to budget energy levels by putting time aside to rest and accomplish the things he wants to accomplish most. Plan activities that require the most energy for times when the energy levels are highest. Encourage the patient to attempt mild aerobic exercise and mild muscle resistance exercise. Do not begin any exercise program without consulting your physician and qualified exercise trainer. It is important to ensure the patient does not have anemia or other problems contributing to the fatigue.

At home, encourage the patient to:

- Allow family, friends, and co-workers to help manage activities.

- Take on small tasks at one time.

- Ask someone else to do the grocery shopping or other errands.

- Ask for help with the children.

- Ask the children to help with chores.

- Plan ahead for cooking and prepare simple meals.

At work, encourage the patient to:

- Think about ways to make work less tiring.

- Ask co-workers to help with some of the work.

- Take regular breaks.

- Park close to the workplace or have someone drop the patient off.

- Ask boss to lighten the workload for awhile.

Nausea and Vomiting

Nausea and vomiting are two common side effects of cancer treatment. Nausea can be immediate and begin a few minutes after a treatment such as chemotherapy and last a short period of time. Less often, it can be delayed and begin two to three days after treatment. This timing varies by patient and depends on the type of chemotherapy treatment given. Some patients may even become physically ill in anticipation of having chemotherapy. Nausea can also be caused by some pain medicine. The causes of nausea can be many in number and complicated.

Unlike many years ago, there are very good medications available today to control both nausea and vomiting caused by cancer and its treatment. Patients who are experiencing these symptoms should talk to their doctors and nurses immediately to get help. While these symptoms may be caused by the treatment, they can also be due to other changes in the body that can accompany cancer. You and the patient should ask the health care team what is causing the nausea.

In addition to medication, a change in eating patterns can sometimes help to alleviate these symptoms as well. Eating several small meals throughout the day may be helpful. Patients who become nauseous during chemotherapy may find that refraining from eating at least two hours before treatment is helpful. Simple relaxation techniques or taking part in relaxing activities are also commonly used to alleviate nausea.

Loss-of-Appetite
Loss-of-appetite is a common symptom that affects people fighting cancer. This can occur when cancer is first diagnosed, and most likely is due to stress and anxiety during chemotherapy or radiation. Advanced stages of cancer can also cause loss-of-appetite. Chronic

nausea often suppresses one's appetite. Chemotherapy can temporarily decrease the patient's ability to taste food. This is another factor that may interfere with appetite.Cancer patients have many challenges in getting proper nutrition.

It is very important that patients continue to eat during treatment in order to keep up strength and maintain nutrition to fight the cancer. Progressive weight loss, anorexia, weakness, exhaustion, lower resistance to infection, problems tolerating cancer treatment, and even death can occur if the patient is not eating properly. Encourage the patient to eat as best as possible under the circumstances.

There are some specific medications that can also be prescribed by your physician that can stimulate appetite. These include some hormones, anabolic steroids, and medicines active in the central nervous system. While these medicines are safe when used as directed, it is very important that your cancer care team supervises them.

Supplements such as "Ensure" or "Boost", which are readily available at most grocery and drug stores, may help.

"Chemo Brain"
Over the years cancer survivors have felt that after

cancer treatment they had problems with memory, concentration, and "knowing the word but not able to think of it". Recent research has validated these reports. Some researchers report that breast cancer patients are more susceptible. Some patients do not experience any changes. These deficits appear to be mild, but it is not yet clear how long they last or what causes them. This is currently a very active area of research, and ways to prevent the deficits are being studied. There is wide agreement among cancer experts that the clear survival advantage of treatment outweighs the risk of this side effect. No one should avoid treatment because of potential "chemo brain" side effects. Again, these problems are manageable, and it is good to be aware of them should problems arise.

Alternative and Complementary Medicine
Alternative and complementary medicine can be defined as treatments that are not widely recognized by medical schools and hospitals in the U.S. These can include chiropractic interventions, acupuncture, massage therapy, nutritional or herbal substances, and homeopathic medicine. Alternative therapies are usually viewed as treatments to be used instead of conventional treatments. Complementary therapies are generally given in addition to conventional cancer treatments. Many alternative and complementary therapies received their roots from Eastern culture and traditions.

Alternative and complementary therapies have grown in popularity over the last 20 years in the United States but continue to conflict with the beliefs of many physicians. While several of these substances are marketed to the public as "natural substances", think of this. Hemlock and tobacco are also "natural substances" – yet it has been scientifically proven that they are harmful to human beings. Many doctors do not believe there is valid scientific evidence that these therapies are safe and effective. There is also concern that some of these therapies may actually be harmful.

It is important to remember that legitimate pharmaceutical medications are regulated by the government and previously approved by the FDA (Food and Drug Administration). Alternative and complementary therapies are not regulated by any governing body nor are they approved by the FDA. The Dietary Supplement Health and Education Act of 1994 limited the role of the FDA and deregulated the herb and dietary supplements industry. Prescription medications are held to a higher standard of purity and effectiveness than are herbal supplements. Animal investigations, clinical trials and post marketing surveillance are not required for herbal supplements.

Additionally, when patients go to the drug store pharmacy to get a physician-prescribed prescription, these medications, along with the patient's personal information, are entered into a relational computer database by the pharmacist. Each time a new medication is prescribed and purchased for that patient, the pharmacist checks this database for potential interactions between various drugs. This information is passed on to the patient for safety purposes. Alternative and complementary therapies are *not* contained in this database, therefore, interactions between these and other drugs are not available.

Getting Alternative and Complementary Advice

If the patient is interested in exploring these types of treatments, all members of the health care team should be consulted. Therapies such as relaxation, massage, aromatherapy, healing touch, acupuncture, hypnosis, and visualization may work well for some patients. Dietary supplements or nutritional regimes, however, should be discussed in detail with the doctors and nurses.

Some alternative and complementary therapies may have very dangerous or adverse effects on cancer treatment and other medications the patient is taking. During the initial visit to the oncologist, the patient should list *all* and *any* alternative/complementary therapies he is taking when filling out the initial paperwork. This is especially important in children, because they react very differently to medications than adults.

A FAMILY MEMBER'S PERSPECTIVE

Judy's mother was diagnosed with terminal lung cancer. Seventy-seven days later, she passed away.

"Things happened so fast. As I look back on it seven years later, I am amazed by how many experiences were compressed into less than three months. Mother had been feeling bad since summer. She kept complaining about pain in her mouth. She went to the dentist, to an infectious disease specialist, and to an otolaryngologist, and no one could figure out what was wrong. All this time she was losing weight, but we never put it together. Then she had a routine chest x-ray and they discovered the mass. Further testing revealed another tumor in her left maxillary sinus – that is where all the mouth pain was coming from all summer and fall. It was decided to treat her with radiation for pain control only. The treatment did not cause any hair loss, but it did cause some superficial burning on her skin. The biggest thing was that it destroyed her appetite.

"She lost so much weight so fast. She would not eat — she just kept saying she wasn't hungry. I kept taking all her favorite foods to her, both at the hospital and at home — milkshakes, Chinese food, pizza, beef and noodles — anything to encourage her to eat. However, no matter what, she just would not eat. I remember

going to the hospital one day and she was sitting on the edge of her bed with her back to the door. Her hospital gown was gaping open in the back, and I was shocked by how prominent her spine and ribs were. That was the first time I really understood how fast she was losing weight.

"I remember complaining to her doctor that she was going to starve to death before the cancer took her. I just could not understand why he would not give her something to increase her appetite so she would eat and get some strength back.

"She lost so much weight in the hospital that she lost her dentures somehow. They had gotten loose, so I think they probably fell out of her mouth during the night and ended up in the hospital laundry. She was so embarrassed to be without her dentures that I found a dentist who would do "same day" dentures. So, we put her in an ambulance, delivered her to the dentist, had her impressions made and took her back to get her dentures the next morning. Besides her self-esteem, I kept thinking she would never be able to eat, even if she wanted to, without her dentures. Of course, the dentures did not matter but it made both of us feel better.

She lost her glasses too, because they were too big so I found an optometrist who would come to the hospital and examine her so we could get new glasses made that fit her face. She was just so emaciated that nothing – clothes, teeth, or even glasses, fit anymore.

"The day I picked her up and took her home from the hospital for hospice care at home, she was so weak she could not walk up the sidewalk to her own front door. As I helped her out of the car, she just kind of sat down on the sidewalk. She could not stand up and I could not pick her up. I was panicked and had no idea what to do. Then a kind man I didn't even know was driving down the street saw us, stopped his car, got out and came over and lifted her up and carried her into the house.

"Once she had the morphine pump at home, she really never ate again, but, by then, it really didn't matter. She was comfortable, there were no more radiation treatments, and the end was near."

HOPE

CHAPTER 5
COPING WITH PHYSICAL CHANGES

Chemotherapy, hormone therapy, immunotherapy, and radiation treatment can cause a lot of changes in the body. While these treatments may kill the cancerous cells, they may also affect the normal cells in the body at the same time, causing some physical changes to occur in the patient. Here are a few of the most common.

Hair Loss
Chemotherapy works by attacking cancerous cells and stopping their growth. Unfortunately, good cells, such as hair follicles, can also be affected and destroyed.

Hair loss occurs in many cancer patients who undergo radiation and certain types of chemotherapy. This typically begins within three to four treatments. The extent of the hair loss is different with each patient and depends upon the type of treatment. Some patients experience mild thinning of the hair, while others lose all their hair. Loss from the eyebrows, eyelashes, underarm, pubic and leg/forearm areas can also occur.

While this side effect is very traumatic for most people, hair usually grows back after treatment is completed – and sometimes even before treatment is over.

Some people who lose all or most of their hair wear turbans, scarves, caps, wigs, or hairpieces. Others leave their head totally uncovered. Patients should be encouraged to do whatever makes them comfortable. Many times, hospitals and clinics have access to local programs that provide self-image counseling for cancer patients as well as wigs and decorative coverings for the head. Patients should ask their oncology nurse for help if they are interested.

Sexuality and Fertility

Cancer and its treatment can have a direct effect on sexuality and fertility. It is not unusual for sexually active people to encounter difficulties and challenges in their sexual lives both during and after cancer treatment. Sexual urges, desires, and even the body's organs themselves can be affected by treatment. Even if the changes are temporary, these changes should be discussed with a member of the patient's health care team the patient is comfortable talking to. That way, the doctor or nurse can refer the patient to a counseling or treatment specialist if unable to answer all the questions.

It is difficult to say how cancer and its treatment will affect a patient's sexuality. Everyone is different. For most, there are changes and challenges that may require some modifications in sexual habits. Cancer can affect the ability to give and receive sexual pleasure, personal body image, feelings, and relationship roles. Patients should keep in mind that these are all intertwined and can all affect one another.

Women can experience symptoms of false menopause such as hot flashes, vaginal itching and dryness, decreased sexual interest, and irregular menstrual periods due to hormone imbalance. Men may also experience hot flashes, as well as infertility, decreased sexual interest, and reduced or damaged sperm cells.

Several factors play a role in this. For instance, chemotherapy, painkillers, anti-depressants, emotional stress from being sick, anxiety, and depression can also reduce sexual desire and interfere with sexual arousal and function.

Because sexuality is such a personal thing, many patients and their spouses find it difficult to discuss sexual issues. In order to maintain a healthy attitude and sexual relationship, however, it is important to discuss them. Patients should let their partner know how they are feeling about participating in sexual activity. Sometimes decreased sexual interest or performance is temporary. The patient's sexual functioning will vary with time. If they don't feel interested in sex, an explanation can help the other partner understand what is happening. Open communication is the best way to deal with sexuality during this time. Asking members of the health care team at the beginning of treatment about expectations relative to sexuality changes may help relieve some of the anxiety for both the patient and the spouse or significant other.

Fluctuations in Weight

The impact of stress, anxiety, depression, and fear of cancer can affect appetite in various ways. The type of treatment a patient undergoes has an impact on appetite as well. For instance, surgery patients often do not feel like eating, however, their body's nutritional needs increase after surgery to help the body to heal.

During radiation therapy, a certain number of "good" cells are destroyed along with the cancerous cells. Depending on what part of the body receives the radiation, some functions of the digestive track can be affected which, in turn, affect a patient's ability to eat.

Chemotherapy may cause nausea, vomiting, and a change in the taste of foods. For these reasons, many patients do not feel like eating during treatment.

Some patients undergoing cancer treatment experience weight gain. It is not readily known what causes this, but intense food cravings may develop in spite of the nausea patients can experience. Patients should eat whatever they want as long as their diet includes a well-balanced intake of foods. Dieting during treatment is not encouraged.

On the opposite side of the spectrum, there are patients who have a poor appetite due to depression or anxiety from cancer treatment. Known as secondary anorexia, patients who experience this are encouraged to eat healthy meals low in fat and high in complex carbohydrates, along with adequate protein. Often times, this will further stimulate the appetite. There are also prescription medications available to help stimulate the appetite.

A PATIENT'S PERSPECTIVE

Mary Jane is 48 years old and fighting a recurrence of breast cancer. More than five years ago she had a mastectomy and thought she had beaten it. Now, she is on chemotherapy again and is struggling with some of the same physical symptoms as before.

"I looked the other day and decided I am going to need a new wig. I thought I would wear the old one this time but it looks pretty shabby. It seems funny now that I didn't throw it away the last time.

"You know, I knew I had cancer again. I can't explain it but I just felt I did. There was something about the way I felt physically – I can't put my finger on exactly what it was but I knew the cancer was back. I put off going to the doctor. Maybe I thought I knew what the treatment was going to be and was dreading it.

"The interesting thing is that my side effects are different this time. I think I am going to lose my hair, but I am not as nauseated this time. The biggest problem I have is that I seem "foggy" at times. I am forgetful and I don't know if it is the chemo or the stress or just plain old age.

"Some days I am so tired I really don't think I can get out of bed. But with two teenagers, it's not easy to stay in bed, so I get up and do what I have to do. But it is a struggle.

"Fortunately, I haven't really lost any weight and I am eating well. When I go back in to see the doctor next time I will tell him about being so tired and about the fogginess. My husband says maybe he can give me something to help. I thought it would get better but it hasn't so I guess I should tell him."

CHAPTER 6
DEATH AND DYING

Talking about Death

"In my experience I find the truth dawns gradually on many, even most of the dying, even when they do not ask and are not told. They accept it quietly, often gratefully, but some may not wish to discuss it, and we must respect their reticence. "

> – Dame Cicely Saunders, founder of
> the hospice movement.

Despite all the advances made in cancer care, sadly, some patients still die. You and the patient should discuss the prognosis with doctors when the time is right to determine if the cancer is potentially life ending. If it is, preparations for end-of-life should begin. That does not mean you, or the patient, are giving up. What it does mean, however, is that you will take care of all those things that need to be taken care of so that you and the patient will be able to focus on the time that is left to live.

Elisabeth Kubler Ross identified five stages the dying patient goes through before death:

Denial
Anger
Bargaining
Depression
Acceptance

Family and caregivers often experience these same stages. At first, there is denial of the diagnosis — the doctor must be wrong. Then, anger sets in — the "why us" response. You may try to bargain with your God: "don't let him die and I will be a better spouse". It is also not unusual, and in fact is very common, for a close family member or caregiver to experience some depression or depressive symptoms. Finally, the illness is accepted — the time you are ready to mentally and emotionally let go of the person you love.

If the person you are caring for is dying, you may find it hard to talk about death and dying. Sometimes the patient has difficulty and is not ready to talk about death either. Other times the family may not want to contemplate the death of the person they love. Often, family and patients try to protect each other from the truth; although both parties usually already know what is happening. You can be helpful to the patient by providing support, comfort and love. Sometimes words are not necessary — your presence alone will provide much comfort. Other times, your willingness to help with the practical challenges of illness, such as running errands, will demonstrate your concern.

Legal Issues

There are many things the patient and family should consider when faced with a terminal illness. Here are just a few: Is there an up-to-date will? Are financial affairs in order — should someone else be authorized to sign checks? Is there a Living Will and does the doctor have a copy? Is there a Health Care Power of Attorney in place? Is there a Durable Power of Attorney? How, and where, does the patient wish to spend his final days? Is hospice care an option? While these can be difficult questions, it is best if the patient and family can discuss these issues openly and honestly. Contact an attorney for help with these items or any legal issues.

Hospice

Many times, much of the pain and anxiety associated with dying can be alleviated by hospice care. Hospice is a concept, not a place. The word comes from the Latin "hospitium," a shelter for weary and sick travelers. Hospice is a philosophy of care focused on easing the physical and emotional pain associated with terminal illness through palliative treatment when a cure is not possible. This is the time when the health care professionals' attention focuses on symptom management and patient comfort. Some patients receive hospice care in a hospice facility. Others receive hospice care at home. Many people want to die at home. No matter where the patient chooses to spend the final days, hospice care will place the emphasis on controlling pain and providing emotional support to both the patient and the family.

The Medicare program includes a hospice benefit that provides coverage for a variety of services and products. Hospice care has been reimbursable under the Medicare Part A benefits option since 1983. As with other services, payment is made on a fixed payment per day that is set by Medicare. Generally speaking, the Medicare hospice benefit is intended primarily for use with patients who have six months or less to live. Doctors may certify a patient for hospice care for two initial 90-day periods of care, followed by an unlimited number of 60-day periods of care. It is important to understand that, under Medicare, a patient may no longer receive active treatment for the cancer if he is to receive hospice benefits. In many states, Medicaid also covers hospice care. Check the patient's health insurance policy to determine any provision for hospice care.

End of Life
Often patients and family members alike want to know what to expect at the end. While no two patients are

alike, there are several common experiences. If the patient is to die of his cancer, the cancer eventually takes control and will leave the patient with little to no energy to fight the illness. He will typically begin to lose weight and may lose an appetite for even his most favorite foods. Sleep becomes more frequent and the patient gradually becomes weaker. Sometimes, the patient will become confused, not recognize loved ones, and even experience hallucinations. Many cancer patients are unconscious when they die, however, they may be able to hear those around them, be aware of their presence, and be reassured by that.

If the patient's faith involves certain end-of-life rituals, it is important that you try to help him attain those rituals. Such rituals may be a great source of comfort.

Dealing with Death
After a loved one dies, people need time to absorb what has happened. If you wish, you may sit with the patient by the bedside for a time. Do whatever your heart tells you. There is no right or wrong way to respond.

Do not be afraid to show your emotions. It is okay to cry, and tears can be a release. It is natural to feel grief when someone you love dies. You may feel physically ill or anxious. You may feel numb or even angry. You may feel guilty, as if there were more you could have done. Some survivors feel depressed. Generally, however, there is a gradual recovery from the acute grief you will feel.

If a funeral is held, some people will continue to offer you support after that occurs. Eventually though, those friends and family move on to their daily lives. This can be the hardest time for family and caregivers, so it's important to take time to focus on yourself and your needs.

There are many grief support groups that you can attend to talk with people in your situation. For example, some communities have widows support groups and support groups for parents of children who have died. You should be able to locate a support group that can serve as a sounding board. (see chapter 12)

The grief process is different for everyone but if you feel unable to cope or if your grief is still significantly interfering with your life after a year, you may want to seek professional counseling. Eventually, you will find a comfortable place for your grief and will be able to "move on" with the memories of your loved one always in your heart.

A FAMILY'S PERSPECTIVE

Jill's 19-year-old son, Craig, was a college freshman when he was diagnosed with a very rare form of cancer.

"He just passed out walking up a set of stairs. His friends took him to the emergency room where the doctors began running tests to determine the cause of the fainting spell. One test revealed a mass in his left atrium.

"He was scheduled for surgery immediately. The cardiologist who did the surgery came in to the waiting room and said, 'well, he made it through the surgery but that's the last good thing I have to say.' He went on to tell us that he was not able to get all the mass and he believed it was cancer. We were all shocked and we remained hopeful that the biopsy would be negative.

"When the biopsy came back it was bad. My husband and I and Craig's 16-year-old brother, Matt, got the news together. Then we went to Craig's room and I was the one who told him. I said, 'you know that tumor they took out—it was cancer.' Craig could not believe it and that was the hardest thing I ever had to say.

"Matt was just devastated. He was very supportive of Craig and he spent a lot of time with him. I remember once Craig told me he could not wait for Matt to grow

up so they could be friends. Matt, being the youngest, was always the baby of the family, but he did grow up overnight. He became very introspective although he still needed and wanted attention from his parents.

"We decided to take Craig to Houston for treatment. For six months either my husband or I was in Houston with Craig at all times. Sometimes, both of us were away, and Matt had to stay with friends, and he hated it; he wanted to stay home alone. I do know he talked to his friends about what was happening with his brother. I don't think he wanted to burden his dad and me. I know at time Matt felt we were giving him less of ourselves than we were giving Craig; but we did not have a choice.

"Before Craig was diagnosed he had already begun to pull away from us. He was a freshman in college and he wanted to be independent. Even when we were in Houston, he wished he could be there alone but his father and I knew we had to be with him.

"Craig went into remission for a few months but it didn't last. On one of his scheduled check-ups, we found out the cancer was back. I think Craig knew he was in trouble before that, because he had been coughing up a lot of blood. But, he was very stoic.

When the doctor told us it was back, Craig asked, 'Am I going to die from this?' The doctor said, 'yes.'

"Now that Craig is gone, we are different as a family. We are more protective of Matt than we would have been had we not lost Craig, but I think Matt understands our fears.

"We are a sadder family now. A lot of people avoid us; we are every parent's nightmare. When it first happened, everyone wanted to help but then, in a while, they moved on. That's normal, so people going through what we did need to find a support group. It is very comforting to talk to someone who really knows how you feel."

CHAPTER 7
SPIRITUALITY AND CANCER

A life-threatening illness such as cancer causes us to confront reality and step back and reflect on our life. It challenges us to look at our anchors. Seeking strength from faith or religion may provide some patients with a perspective that can help them deal with the issues of disease and with emotions that face them.

Our Mortality

The diagnosis of cancer or other serious illnesses confronts us with our mortality and our limited time on this earth. When fighting for their lives, patients often reflect on their ultimate priorities and think about what they truly want in their lives. Patients may talk of surviving for the sake of their family members, or to meet certain life goals they had. Whatever the reasons, this can be reflected by religious, spiritual, or philosophical beliefs about what is important in their lives and why.

While many cancer patients may have feelings of regret

that it took a serious illness to get their attention, many positive changes can also result.

Why Me?

Cancer and other serious illnesses force us to ask the question "why". Why did this have to happen to me? One reason for this may be religious in nature. For those who believe in the God of the Judeo-Christian Bible, they sometimes do not understand how such a God could allow cancer to happen to a good person.

While most religions today reject the idea that God punishes us through illness, some patients may ask themselves if they are being punished for wrongdoing or failings of character. Others, however, may feel that their illness is part of God's overall life journey for them. Even patients who are not particularly religious may feel a sense of self-blame about their cancer. The "why me" question is an emotional reaction to the overwhelming issues patients face with a life threatening illness. For some people, religion and spirituality provides comfort and reassurance.

Religion, Faith, and Spirituality

For cancer patients, many questions may arise about religion, faith, and spirituality. Religion is the formal study of belief and the organized understanding of beliefs shared by groups of people. Faith often refers to beliefs held by an individual who practices one of the formal systems of religion and may form a foundation of emotional and spiritual strength when we face crisis – especially death. Spirituality can be defined as a connection many people feel to their God or to something beyond this world. Many people speak about being spiritual but not necessarily religious.

Coping and Healing

Faith and spirituality can provide an avenue to cope with illness and reach an inner healing. Coping can mean different things to different patients. Some may find that religion will enable them cope with their illness. It may provide a community of believers that can provide support. It may provide answers. It may give comfort. It may alleviate fears. It may help the patients to bring their values in line with their religious or spiritual beliefs. This process is different for everyone. As a caregiver, if you are not affiliated with a specific religion or faith, you should still encourage the patient to participate in his. It may be an extra anchor to carry him through the illness. If the patient is not religious and has no particular faith, it should not be forced upon him to change his beliefs. Spirituality and religion are very personal decisions and should be respected as such.

Spirituality and Qualify-of-Life

More and more, questions are being raised as to whether spirituality is a legitimate part of treatment. Some research studies have revealed that a rich spiritual life may improve patient outcomes and their quality-of-life. Techniques such as visualization, meditation, and prayer are being utilized more and more in the medical community as coping mechanisms for patients. Healing touch may provide "healing relief" that is different from the concept of "cure." Some teaching institutions believe that religious or spiritual practices have an impact on physical and mental health, on the meaning a particular illness has for people, and on the decisions patients make about seeking health care. Religion may also be used as a way for coping with health-related stress. This trend is becoming so strong that many medical schools in the United States are now offering spirituality and medicine courses as part of their curriculum.

A PATIENT'S PERSPECTIVE

Carol was 54 years old when she learned she had bladder cancer. Then, just two weeks later, the doctors told her she had Hodgkin's disease. Her bladder cancer was quickly in remission and then, two years later she had a recurrence of the bladder cancer. In another year, she learned she now had non-Hodgkin's Lymphoma. While she has had four battles with cancer in three years, Carol never questions why.

"It was difficult for me to believe I had cancer the first time. There was no family history of cancer. Then, when they told me two weeks later I had Hodgkin's disease, I had to believe it. The fourth time I had cancer they told me I only had a 50% chance of survival but I am still here and I beat it. Once they thought I might have lung cancer, too but I just prayed and I believe the power of prayer kept lung cancer from coming.

"I never said, why me. I have no fear of death. My attitude is that I will always beat cancer – or I will go home to my Lord, but cancer won't beat me.

"Sometimes I wonder, how do I survive and other people get cancer and die? I think it is faith. I never pray for a cure, I pray to God for the strength to handle whatever comes my way. I believe if you ask

God for help, he will help you. It may not be in the way you ask, but he will help. I think if someone has a marginal faith, they will develop a strong faith when they get cancer.

"*I tell people you need four things to survive cancer: dedicated doctors, good medicine, the power of prayer, and the grace of God. If you have all four of these working for you, you are really fortunate.*"

A CLERGYMAN'S PERSPECTIVE

Gordon has been a hospital chaplain for fifteen years. During that time he has seen many cancer patients. Some survived and some did not. But, he is certain there is a difference between the way a person with faith deals with a life-threatening disease and the way a person who does not have a faith base reacts. He also sometimes sees differences in the way the patient and his family approach cancer depending upon their faith.

"*There is no question at all that if a person has a faith system or a belief system, he has a source of emotional and spiritual support that others do not. The deeper the level of commitment to the faith, the more strength that can be drawn.*

"*I work with end-of-life patients and those with faith*

don't seem to suffer with the outcome as much. Every patient asks 'why me' at first. But, as the treatment progresses, the person who is a believer seems to accept it more quickly.

"The cancer patient may have a belief system that allows him to find strength and hope but, sometimes the family doesn't share that system and there is nothing for them to cling to. In other cases, the family may have a strong faith and be very vocal about it while the patient seems less devout.

"Families must realize that salvation and peace with God is a very personal matter and each person must be allowed to act as he wishes. Quiet, private faith is just as strong as faith that is more vocal.

"I believe the chaplains' role is:
- *To simply be there – a ministry of presence*
- *To pray – sometimes people don't feel comfortable praying on their own*
- *To perform rituals – communion, baptisms, holy sacraments, etc.*

"Families and patients should contact us directly or ask the doctor or nurse to make a referral if they feel we can help them. We may not be needed for all three of our roles, but we are ready to do whatever we can to ease the way of the patient and family."

CHAPTER 8
ILLNESS AND FAMILY RELATIONSHIPS

Sometimes patients have problems changing roles – especially if they have been very active or served in the role as the primary caregiver of the family. Those people who have been the most active caregivers have the hardest time asking for help. Almost always, one or more family members or friends take over some or all of the duties – at least temporarily – of the patient. Roles begin to change. Roles may begin to reverse. Routines become disrupted. It affects everyone including the person with the illness. People handle stressful situations and cope with illness in very different ways. As we discussed in chapter one, the 5D's (death, dependence, disruption, disability, and disfigurement) are emotional markers that can influence family relationships.

A good starting point to understanding and dealing with these emotions and interactions is to get the patient and family members on the same page at the beginning of the illness. Gathering accurate information, becoming educated about the illness, and understanding what to expect from the treatment and illness itself is important.

Role Changes

Almost invariably, roles change when a family member is diagnosed with cancer. Usually, someone in the family will take over the duties of the patient who is ill. This can cause anxiety, anger, and eventually depression on the part of the patient because he may feel more dependent upon – and sometimes even a burden on – other family members. For a sick person, giving up daily roles can be an enormous loss. As a caregiver, understanding this from the beginning of the illness is important.

Parenting the Parent

Even the best functioning families are affected by cancer. When the caregiver is the son or daughter and the patient is the parent, the dynamics can become very complicated. Roles are now reversed. The balance of power shifts. The parent is now the "child", and the child becomes the "parent". Subtle and complex changes take place in relationships between parents and children as they grow older. While the parents were responsible for the children for many years, now the son or daughter is being called upon to ensure the care and welfare of the parent. In these situations, sons and daughters can find themselves caught between respecting their parents' right to remain independent and knowing when to step in and help.

As a caregiver, the more you are able to make decisions *with* a parent, the better you will both be. When in doubt of your decisions, seek the input of other relatives, friends, and members of your health care team. They may be able to give you some objective input.

Disruption of Routines and Relationships
Inevitably, family routines are also disrupted – at least for a period of time – during an illness. There can be numerous doctor's appointments, lab tests, treatment schedules, hospital visits, and other tasks that need to be done. The demands of the illness can affect the entire family. Schedules will change, and everyone will need to pitch in. The best thing to remember is to be flexible. Special attention should be paid to children who are involved because disruption is especially difficult on them.

Many times, tragedy can bring family members closer together. If not managed properly, however, it can also cause people to withdraw and grow apart. Many times, family members have a sense of helplessness because they do not know what to say to their loved one or how to help them through the illness.

Helping Your Children Cope With the Illness

When illness strikes families with children, communication becomes especially important. Children are smart and can usually perceive that something is wrong. Providing them with an honest explanation about the illness will help them cope with the situation in a healthy way. Helping young people adapt properly to a family illness will influence how they deal with other difficult situations in their future. Communication is not a one-time event, rather a very important ongoing process that will need to continue throughout the course of the illness and beyond.

Assigning children small tasks to help can make them feel involved in and part of the process. Older children can take on bigger responsibilities such as cooking, helping to care for the younger children in the family, or running errands.

When Your Child is the Patient

Childhood cancers are typically categorized as solid tumors, lymphomas, and leukemias. These cancers are usually fast growing, but often respond well to treatment. Childhood cancers are treated similarly to adult cancers – with surgery, chemotherapy, and radiation. Because children are still in the growth and development phases of their lives, treatment can often be strenuous, difficult, overwhelming, and emotionally painful.

When children have to undergo treatment without a total understanding for the need, they may become anxious and develop behavioral problems. A common reaction of seriously ill children is to regress to a seemingly younger age. Behavior and habits that were seen when the child was younger may re-appear. The way a parent reacts to the illness and treatment has a direct influence on child's ability to cope. Talking with the care team to learn what to expect and how to respond is important. Learning coping skills such as behavioral techniques can be useful to reduce the pain and anxiety that the child is experiencing. If the child is in school, proactive communication with the teachers and classmates will be critical. Setting the stage properly can have an impact on how the child will be treated, especially by his peers. Decide what you want people to know about the illness, and communicate that openly and honestly. Encourage schoolmates to ask questions.

If you do not feel that your child is coping well or if you have questions, an early consultation with a professional who understands childrens' reactions to illness is very important. A social worker or professional in pediatric behavior can also provide guidance for these issues.

Keeping Lines of Communication Open
Talking and *listening* to one another is an important component in dealing with an illness. Some patients

may not want to acknowledge they are ill, and therefore, will not want to talk about their cancer. This may be in conflict with family members who want to discuss the illness and get their feelings and fears out in the open. Other patients may be more open and willing to discuss their disease, progress and treatments. At the same time, their family members may be trying to manage their own fears and anxieties and unable to communicate with the patient.

These issues are often the cause of miscommunication. Having the courage to discuss the fears and concerns of illness is very important in the communications process. Holding regular family meetings where every member gets a turn to talk and discuss their feelings and concerns can be helpful.

Seeking help from professionals — members of your oncology team, psychiatrists, psychologists, and social workers — is also beneficial. They can facilitate objective communication and provide relief to patients and family members during an illness.

TWO PATIENTS' PERSPECTIVES

Patricia is a cancer survivor who is caring for her 92-year-old mother who suffers from multiple health problems. The situation is becoming more and more difficult as time goes on. Pat feels enormous pressure caring for her mother and does not like the role in which she finds herself.

"I was just looking at my calendar. I have taken her to 39 doctor's appointments so far this year. I go there every Sunday after church to visit. I worry about how much longer she can live in her apartment. It's terrible. Instead of being friends with her, I am now the mother. She doesn't want to hear my suggestions and so we end up bickering. I hate it. I go away from seeing her and I cry part of the way home. I feel like I should be giving her more comfort, and instead I am doing the mothering."

Judy's mother died less than three months after being diagnosed with lung cancer. As the oldest child, she found herself in the position of decision-maker and advisor for her mother.

"She began to lean on me very soon after her diagnosis. She knew from the beginning that her prognosis was poor. I think she was overwhelmed and wanted to hand

over the decision-making to someone else. As the oldest child, it was natural for me to take over. I was lucky as, mother had made her wishes known to all of us. She had a living will and a health care power of attorney. All I had to do was to follow what I knew she wanted. There was a time, during the first few weeks when I could sense she was angry about what was happening to her. One day she lashed out at me for no reason. I answered back, 'Don't yell at me; it's not my fault you have cancer.'

"Those were the only cross words we ever exchanged. It was hard to watch her fade away, but in some ways it was comforting to be able to care for her the way she had cared for us for so many years. I remember her telling a friend that 'the kids have been so good to me.' Of course, we were good to her. We were just paying back all that love and nurturing she had given us. I considered it a privilege to help care for her."

CHAPTER 9
WORKPLACE CHALLENGES

According to the American Cancer Society, cancer rates continue to fall in the U.S., but the actual number of cancer patients will double by 2050. The number of newly diagnosed patients can be expected to rise from 1.3 million to 2.6 million people. Because of the advances in the management of cancer's side effects over the last several years, more people living with cancer are able to work while receiving their treatment. In today's society, work provides not only monetary support, but also a person's identity and sense of self-worth.

After a patient finishes cancer treatment, he often expects to return to a "normal" way of life, including going back to work. Everyone reacts differently to this situation. Some people are ready to "jump right back in." Others are hesitant, but it is their financial means of support, so they may feel there is no other choice. For others, priorities may have changed in their lives, and work may no longer be the focal point. As a caregiver, it is important to help encourage the patient to ease back into this in a way that is comfortable for him.

Workplace Performance

Sometimes, employers may not fully understand the effect cancer has had on their employee. Patients may experience both physical and emotional side effects of cancer and its treatment, and these may affect their performance at work.

Unfortunately, many myths about cancer still exist in our society, and the workplace is no exception. An employer may assume that a patient can no longer perform the same tasks, or that stress makes him a poor risk for promotion. Co-workers may also believe that they will be required to do extra work because the patient cannot do his job. Employers and co-workers may also see care giving responsibilities as overwhelming, and make these same assumptions. Any or all of these approaches toward people with cancer and/or family members can lead to negative issues in the workplace.

Workplace Challenges

Physical and emotional symptoms can cause challenges for some patients in the workplace. While undergoing treatment, patients may experience symptoms such as fatigue and nausea at work. These can temporarily impact their performance. Talking to the employer before returning to work and asking for some temporary flexibility can be helpful. Requesting flexible hours and duties that are not physically strenuous, as well as asking for help when needed can also make the transition easier.

The ability to return to work should be a happy occasion after an illness, though patients often find themselves facing unexpected challenges. Remember that patients are protected by the Americans with Disabilities Act (ADA). If there is suspicion of discrimination because of their illness, legal remedies are available.

Talking With Co-Workers

To some degree, patients can control the way they are treated when they return to work. The atmosphere set by the patient has a great deal of influence on the reactions of co-workers. It is best to help the patient decide what he wants people to know. Sometimes it is helpful for a patient to plan ahead and have some statements ready when he is asked "How are you?". The patient may also want to have some answers that will gently but firmly say "I don't want to talk about it." If possible, upon returning to work, the patient may want to sit down and talk to his boss — either in a group or private setting — depending on each individual's situation. Tell them as much about the cancer as the patient wants them to know. Encourage employees to ask questions, and be open and honest. Typically, the more open the patient is, the less gossip and speculation there will be.

Caregiver Workplace Challenges
Assuming the role of a caregiver is very time consuming. So often, you are concerned with the well being of the patient that you forget about yourself. If you are acting as the primary caregiver during an illness, be prepared for your schedule to change and become somewhat disrupted. If you work outside of the home, this may also include your daily schedule in the workplace. You need to begin to think about how to handle time away from the office and proper prioritization of your duties with the patient. There are times when it will be especially important for you to be available to help the patient, whether to give emotional support, attend doctor's appointments, or help with other activities. Here are some simple guidelines to think about.

Be available:
At the beginning of the illness when diagnosis takes place.

If there is a change in the treatment the patient is receiving.

If there has been a relapse in the illness.

During treatment cycles when the patient experiences fatigue.

If the patient has expressed he "needs" you.

If the patient is not physically able to drive to treatments or doctor appointments.

Quite often, employers are willing to be flexible for those assuming caregiver responsibilities. That flexibility, depending on the employer, however, may be temporary, so it is best to communicate right away with your boss. Plan ahead as much as possible and provide a schedule of times you anticipate being gone. Offer to make time up where appropriate.

The Family and Medical Leave Act, which became effective in the early 1990s, entitles eligible employees to take up to 12 weeks of unpaid, job-protected leave within a 12-month period for specified family and medical reasons. There are certain criteria for eligibility, so check with your employer for more information and if this might be an option for you to consider.

A PATIENT'S PERSPECTIVE

Susan, a high school guidance counselor, was only 36 years old when she was diagnosed with breast cancer. She continued to work fulltime during her treatment.

"I was working fulltime, directing the school musical, and had a three-year-old at home. I missed very little work. I did miss a few mornings after chemotherapy, but not many. Everyone at work was extremely solicitous and everyone offered to help. The people at school were very nice and patient.

"I did not tell the students, although some knew because their parents knew. If people asked questions, I did talk about it. I would say 'this is just a bump in the road and as long as I live nothing else matters'. People handle things in such dramatically different ways. I just wanted to keep my life as normal as possible and keep busy. I think that helped me maintain some sense of control. I just didn't want to talk about it with everyone; I am not comfortable in that kind of situation."

CHAPTER 10
PAYING FOR CANCER CARE

There is no doubt about it – cancer care is expensive. Cancer treatment can be financially devastating, so information about treatment costs and health insurance particulars need to be discussed at the onset of an illness. Encourage the patient to be honest and open with the doctor about his financial situation. Ask the doctor to provide a relative dollar amount of what the treatments will cost, what will be covered under the insurance policy and what portion will be required to be paid by the patient. That way, financial expectations are set up front and there are no surprises along the way. If the patient does not have health insurance, this should also be addressed with the doctor right away. People without health insurance or inadequate insurance may face barriers to getting the care they need, however, there are assistance programs available to help overcome these barriers.

A good resource to discuss these options is the hospital social worker. He will be knowledgeable about any special financial assistance offered by that particular hospital as well as local or state programs (i.e., state-funded insurance plans) available in the community. Some hospitals receive funding from the federal government to provide free or low-cost care to patients who are unable to pay. This is called Hill-Burton funding. If a patient is without insurance or unable to pay, this may be a potential source of help. Hospitals that accept Medicare and Medicaid are required to comply with Hill-Burton.

Uninsured patients who have limited financial assets may qualify for Medicaid assistance. Talk to the health care team or social worker about this option. If the patient is a veteran, there may also be some additional benefits. Contact the Veterans Administration for further information.

Borrowing against a 401 (k) or other retirement plan may also be an option to pay medical expenses. Patients should discuss this with their human resources representative at their place of employment for specific details. Accessing the benefits of a life insurance policy is another option. Some life insurance companies enable policyholders to access the funds from a policy prior to death. There are also companies called viaticals that will purchase the insurance policy for a discounted amount (which is an amount less than face value). This enables the policyholder to receive cash from the policy to pay for medical and other expenses. If the patient considers this option, the details and fine print should be reviewed very carefully. Seeking the expertise of an accountant or banker is a good resource to help the patient answer questions and make decisions about all of these options.

Paying For Medication
If patients need help paying for prescription medications, many pharmaceutical companies have assistance programs that provide free and discounted medicine to people who cannot afford them. The oncology doctor or nurse can help put the patient in touch with the appropriate contacts for those programs. Some states also have pharmaceutical assistance programs that help pay for the cost of drugs. A hospital social worker can usually help a patient make an application to a program that fits his needs.

A PATIENT'S PERSPECTIVE

Robert Urich was a successful actor in 1996 when he learned he had synovial cell sarcoma. However, despite his financial means, he realized immediately that if he did not alter his lifestyle in some ways, he would not be able to maintain his family without working. In a year 2000 interview, he shared his concerns about the financial challenges of cancer.

"They canceled my TV series, "The Lazarus Man", when they found out I had cancer, and my commercial endorsements dried up. Bills started to mount. I was lucky to have good insurance. But for two years I had to live on almost every penny I had saved in my 25-year career. I can only imagine what other families are faced with. I was lucky. Not everyone has the resources I had. I had more means than most people but even so, I quickly realized what going without any income could do to you. Unfortunately, some people have to make life or death decisions based upon finances."

CHAPTER 11
PARTICIPATING IN RESEARCH AND CLINICAL TRIALS

When you hear the term research, do you wonder what it means and what it entails? Cancer research is conducted through many channels such as the National Cancer Institute, teaching institutions and universities, pharmaceutical companies, hospitals, private medical practices, or other sources. A clinical trial is a research project that a university, government entity, hospital, or other group may conduct to evaluate if a particular treatment process (such as chemotherapy, hormone therapy, radiation, or some combination of these) is effective. Clinical trials are done in different phases or stages, which allow researchers to review specific information about the various treatment processes. Clinical trials compare drug and other treatment regimens.

In the U.S., there are many safeguards for patients who participate in clinical trials. A clinical trial must be approved by what is known as an institutional review board, which serves as a watchdog group to protect the participants. This ensures the trial does not put patients at undue risk. Clinical trials use both active medicines and also what are known as placebos — which are inactive substances. In cancer research, it is highly unlikely that a patient would be given a placebo by itself without other active substances. Any placebo given would be accompanied by active medicine.

How Can a Clinical Trial Benefit a Patient?
There can be many benefits of participation in a clinical trial. First, if the patient's physician is participating in a trial, chances are, he is being treated by a physician who stays abreast of the latest developments in cancer research and is interested in providing up-to-date care for his patients. It also allows the patient to take a proactive role in his health care.

Other benefits include:
- Access to the latest treatments and interventions that are currently available.

- Potentially receiving the newest treatments available at little or no cost.

- Regular monitoring of the patient's health care and condition.

- Contribution to medical knowledge to help other patients.

Is a Clinical Trial Appropriate?

If the patient is interested in participating in a clinical trial, he should talk to the physician and oncology nurse about the details. Patients should take notes about their questions and concerns before talking to the health care team, and should be encouraged to bring a family member along. Here are some important questions to ask:

- What type of study is this and who will sponsor it?

- What are the expectations of the trial?

- How long will the clinical trial last? Who will be monitoring the patient's care during the trial?

- What are the potential benefits and risks/side effects that could affect the patient personally? Will a placebo be used?

- What is the cost involved if any? Will health care insurance cover what is not covered by the trial?

- What will participation in the trial involve? How often will the patient have procedures, receive treatments, etc.?

Answering these questions should give you and the patient a better and more detailed understanding of the specific clinical trial and whether it is appropriate for the patient's individual situation. It is important to know how the trial will benefit the patient and any risks involved. It is also critical to ensure that a reputable group is conducting the trial.

What Happens at the Completion of a Clinical Trial?

When a patient participates in a clinical trial, his information — and that of every participant — will be collected and submitted confidentially to the entity that conducted the trial. Once analyzed, they inform the public of the study results. Most times, results are published in medical or scientific journals. Often, results are communicated via the national news media on television and in newspapers. Once a treatment is proven safe and effective from the outcome of a clinical trial, it may become a new standard of practice and made widely available.

CHAPTER 12
FINDING SUPPORT AND ASKING FOR HELP

Cancer affects everyone close to the patient – even the best functioning families. The problems and emotional issues it creates can be difficult to accept. Many times, families face challenges that leave them feeling afraid and overwhelmed. The support of others, including family members, friends, co-workers, peers, religious contacts, others who have had cancer, or cancer support organizations can help those affected by cancer feel less alone and deal more effectively with their challenges.

What is Support?

Support can take many forms. It may include a person or persons who: regularly takes the patient to doctor appointments/treatment sessions, does the grocery shopping, cleans the house, picks the children up from school, and runs the errands. Or, it may be a more formal support network such as an advocacy group. These more formal support groups give patients, caregivers, loved ones, and other cancer survivors a way to openly and confidentially discuss their problems and fears and cope with their illness along with others who are experiencing similar challenges. Support, both informal and formal, is very important during an illness.

Caregivers Need Support Too

Caregivers, family members and other loved ones can be just as affected by cancer as the patient, and they, too, often need assistance dealing with the issues surrounding disease. For that reason, some support groups have been developed specifically for family members and loved ones. Other support groups encourage family and loved ones to participate along with the cancer patient/survivor.

The Importance of Support

Cancer can cause great stress for both patients and caregivers, family members, and loved ones who care about them. Engaging the help of family and friends as well as formal support groups or networks can help relieve stress and positively impact life. Support can help to relieve stress, whether it's just a family member or friend offering to help with day-to-day household duties, or attending a formal support group meeting. Support can also reduce the feeling of aloneness. When patients are around other people who want to help, whether in a formal or informal setting, the sense of isolation and loneliness may not seem as overwhelming.

Staying connected with others can also improve mood and keep the spirits higher. It is also a way to get more objective practical information about coping strategies.

Using Personal Support Networks Effectively

Friends, family members, colleagues, neighbors, and co-workers are all good examples of informal support. Tapping into these resources may enable patients to feel they can maintain some normalcy in their life during a time when life has been turned upside down. The most important thing to remember, whether a patient, a caregiver, or a family member: don't be afraid to ask members of your support network for help. Family and friends can help in a number of ways, depending on the patient's individual situation. If they are good at specific tasks, take that into consideration when asking for help. Give them specific assignments to do, and let them be a resource to help you.

Formal Support Networks

Formal support groups and networks are typically led and overseen by trained professionals and conducted in a group setting. This can include self-help groups, support groups, therapy and counseling, as well as religious or other organizations. These settings are helpful for exchanging information as well as raising awareness about an illness. Formal support also enables patients, families, caregivers, and loved ones to talk openly and focus on daily adjustment to living with an illness. There are many types of support groups and programs available for patients and families to deal with all phases of cancer care. Some are support groups, while other, more specialized groups may be geared toward children, young adults, or patients/survivors who have a particular type of cancer.

Professionally led support groups are typically organized and run by professionals in a certain field of health care expertise. Self-help groups are usually run by the members, themselves and most times do not involve professional leaders. Both types of groups can be helpful to patients and loved ones, depending on their particular needs and situation.

Finding a Support Group

Many organizations offer support groups for cancer patients and their family members or friends. The health care team is a good resource to inquire about support, especially as it relates to local efforts. Most hospitals have social services departments that can also provide information about cancer support groups and programs. The final chapter of this book provides a listing of cancer resources, including helpful websites and phone numbers.

CHAPTER 13
CANCER AND HEALTHY LIVING

Just because a diagnosis of cancer has been made doesn't mean it is too late! As we discussed earlier, cancer can be a chronic disease rather than an acute one. Good health behaviors remain important and sometimes become even more important after cancer is diagnosed. This is another important aspect of not giving up. We can think of good health behaviors in two general categories: mental and physical.

An important part of healthy living is tending to our "mental health." Sometimes in the press of our daily lives and schedules, personal priorities and personal goals can spin out of control or be lost. Patients sometimes say or feel "...I wish I did not have to have this cancer to know what I know now..." The benefit of a brush with a serious health problem can be a second look at how we are spending our time and how we are treating people around us. Are we spending enough time with loved ones, devoting enough time to helping others or giving enough time to our own personal or spiritual development? These are all questions that may surface when someone confronts a serious health problem. These are topics that your loved one may wish to discuss. If you do not feel comfortable or adequate to work through these issues, some sessions with your pastor, priest, rabbi, or a counselor may be helpful. Spirituality is discussed in more detail in Chapter 7. A take-home message is that these discussions should not be avoided or suppressed.

Tending to our physical health may involve maintaining good nutrition, starting an exercise regimen, and controlling use of substances such as alcohol or nicotine.

The Importance of Proper Nutrition

Both during and after cancer treatment, patients should focus on maintaining their strength and an overall healthy lifestyle. Proper nutrition becomes increasingly important because the impact of stress, anxiety, depression, and fear of cancer can affect appetite in different ways. Good nutritional practices can help cancer patients to maintain their strength and overall well-being. Poor nutrition can contribute to the intensity of treatment side effects as well as cause mal-nutrition and weight loss, increased risk of unrelated illness or infection, and reduced chances for survival. Different types of cancer and cancer treatment affect the appetite in different ways. For instance, nutritional problems can be caused from the effects of a cancerous tumor that is present in the gastrointestinal tract. This can cause digestive problems such as obstruction of the gastrointestinal tract and malabsorption (nutrients are not properly absorbed), nausea, vomiting, and diarrhea. Relative to cancer treatment, **surgery** can cause fatigue, depression, or loss-of-appetite, so many patients are unable to eat for a period of time. If the surgery involves any portion of the mouth or digestive tract, digestion and food absorption can also be temporarily affected. **Chemotherapy** and **immunotherapy** can cause side effects such as nausea, vomiting, and diarrhea, which can diminish the appetite. There are, however, several medications available to control these side effects. Patients who experience these symptoms need to make their health care team aware in order to alleviate the problems. **Radiation therapy** kills cancerous cells, and in the process, may also damage normal cells. If those cells are located in or around areas of the gastrointestinal tract, this may affect a patient's ability to eat. Eating can even become painful.

Patients should be encouraged to eat whatever they want as long as meals include a balanced intake of foods. Dieting during cancer treatment is not recommended. A well-balanced diet, which includes foods that provide the proper amounts of nutrients will help the patient to maintain body weight and continue to fight the cancer. A patient's eating habits should be continually evaluated by the oncology team during the course of the treatment.

Inclusion of the major food groups in the diet every day is an important factor for proper nutrition. These food groups include breads/cereals/grains, vegetables/fruits, meat/poultry/fish, and milk/cheese products. Proper diet also means including foods high in fiber and that provide all the nutrients needed to stay healthy during and after cancer treatment. Essential nutrients include the following:

- **Proteins** stimulate growth, repair body tissue, and keep the immune system functioning properly. Food sources include meat, fish, poultry, milk/cheese products, nuts, and soy products.

- **Carbohydrates and fats** provide the majority of calories for daily activity. Carbohydrate food sources include fruits and vegetables, breads, cereals, and pastas. Sources of fat include oils, nuts, butter, and margarine.

- **Water** prevents dehydration and is essential, especially during cancer treatment.

- **Vitamins and minerals** are important for ongoing growth. A well-balanced diet typically provides adequate vitamins and minerals. If supplements are taken during cancer treatment, however, the health care team should be consulted because these can sometimes interfere with some chemotherapy drugs.

For patients who are faced with an ongoing lack of appetite, a variety of prescription medications are available that help to stimulate the appetite. Again, these options should be discussed with the health care team.

Eating Tips
- Eat several small meals during the day.
- Eat what tastes good.
- Try some of the liquid supplements, such as Ensure, (those that are high in nutrients and calories) or ProSure with a scoop of ice cream or flavored syrup to enhance the taste. Try them after they have been refrigerated.

After Treatment
Most appetite problems and other eating-related symptoms disappear after treatment is completed, however, these can sometimes linger. If this occurs, patients may wish to consult a dietician to help them

plan an ongoing well-balanced diet plan they can follow. Continuing to eat well is important and enables patients to build strength and maintain overall good health. Additionally, dieticians often perform screenings and assessments to determine if other types of professional nutrition therapy may be needed.

Exercise and Fitness

Exercise improves health. Research shows that physical activity and exercise have a positive effect on cancer patients, can improve their quality of life, and help lessen depression. Exercise can improve physical strength, physical stamina, and the ability to combat the side effects of chemotherapy, including nausea and fatigue. It may also have a positive effect on mental and emotional health. While the long-term effects of regular exercise provide positive impacts to improve health, any immediate effects on the immune system are still unknown.

While aerobic exercise keeps the heart and lungs in good working order, weight training can also be beneficial because it maintains muscular strength and endurance, boosts metabolism, and strengthens bones. This is especially important for the prevention of osteo-porosis later in life. Both forms of exercise can be effective in managing fatigue caused by cancer treatment. Interestingly, fatigue caused by illness can be combated by mild exercise. Resting may not diminish the effects of fatigue, however, exercise can provide an energy boost.

How Much Exercise is Enough?
How much exercise depends on several factors. If patients did not exercise prior to cancer treatment, they should begin slowly with more moderate activities and build up their duration per session and frequency throughout the week. Building up to a total of 30 minutes at one time may be a reasonable goal to set for improving the overall fitness level. For patients who were already active, intensity can be increased as they feel comfortable resuming their exercise program. In most cases, less can be more — patients don't necessarily need to set aside long periods of time for exercise to be effective. Exercise can be done two to three times per day in smaller increments (rather than all at once) and still be effective. It all depends on each individual's own fitness level and particular situation. Aerobic exercise is any type of activity that causes your muscles to use oxygen and elevates the heart rate. This can be accomplished through various exercises such as walking outside or on a treadmill, jogging, cycling, swimming, dancing, fitness classes, etc.

It is important to note that no matter what a patient's fitness level is, the oncology team should be consulted

before beginning or re-starting an exercise program. If beginning weight training for the first time, it is also a good idea to consult a certified exercise trainer after getting the green light from the physician.

Starting Slowly

For patients who are new to exercise or experience fatigue from their treatment, here are some tips that will help ease them into activity. Be sure to get the doctor's approval!

- Be sure to stretch the leg muscles before beginning.
- Take the stairs rather than the elevator.
- Bring tennis shoes to work and walk during breaks and lunchtime.
- Go to the shopping mall and walk the inside perimeter several times.
- If you have a dog, take it for a walk every day.
- Find someplace to walk up and down the stairs.
- Mow the lawn.

Alcohol, Nicotine and the Concept of Harm Reduction

In the United States the two most common drugs that cause significant health problems are alcohol and nicotine. Both of these substances are associated with increased incidence of cancer. Both of these substances can interfere with cancer treatment.

Alcohol. Excessive use of alcohol is a term that is hard to define. For discussion here we will use the definition of more than two drinks (each with 1.5 ounces of alcohol), two bottles of beer, or two glasses of wine per day. Excessive use of alcohol has been associated with poor nutrition and poor compliance with treatment. People who are intoxicated often forget to take their medication, go to the doctor, or eat properly. Alcohol is toxic to the liver. Many medications are metabolized by the liver and alcohol may add stress to even a normal liver. Preserving liver function is very important, therefore, reducing alcohol intake is important.

Nicotine. In addition to the harmful, irritating, and cancer-causing effects of the contents of cigarette, cigar, or pipe smoke, nicotine has other harmful effects. Nicotine is the primary agent in tobacco smoke that causes addiction. Nicotine is probably the only drug that will cause very significant harm to our bodies even when we take it in what is considered to be normal amounts, i.e., one pack of cigarettes per day. Nicotine has been associated with increased vascular disease. It prevents surgical incisions from healing. Nicotine can cause significant increases in blood clots. The research evidence for these problems is overwhelming. Additionally, a reduction in tars and other pollutants in tobacco smoke is very beneficial. Stopping nicotine use is very important actually, whether one has cancer or not.

The concept of harm reduction. Both alcohol and nicotine can cause very strong addiction (see Chapter 4). It may be difficult or impossible to stop use of these substances; however, many of the negative effects of these substances are dose related. That means, even if one cannot quit using, reducing the amount may be helpful. This does not mean that a person who has no control over use of alcohol or is in a recovery program should try to drink more moderately. It does, however, mean that for those people who abuse these substances, using less can have a very positive impact on their health. It is worth the trouble to work with the health care team to reduce consumption. It is all about cultivating and growing good health behaviors.

A PATIENT'S PERSPECTIVE

Constance was shocked by her cancer diagnosis. She was never one to pay much attention to her health, so the fact that she was ill with a life-threatening disease was something she had never anticipated. Never one to eat healthy or exercise, having cancer changed her views on a healthy life style.

"I don't know if my lousy health habits had anything to do with getting cancer, but as soon as I found out, I started changing a lot of things. The first thing I did was lay off the junk food. I started eating healthy; lots of vegetables and fruits and more chicken and fish than I had been used to eating. No more big steaks. The other thing I did was start exercising. First, I just started walking around my neighborhood and pretty soon I was walking a bit farther. Some good friends have a swimming pool and let me swim in their pool every day I felt like it. I wasn't swimming fast laps, mind you, but it did make me feel better.

"Now that the cancer is gone I am still following a healthy diet. I walk every day and I have even walked in some fundraising walks for charity. I don't know for sure, but I think changing my health habits may have helped me fight my cancer. I am thinking about joining a gym or going to a personal trainer now that I am well."

CHAPTER 14
RESOURCES

The Internet – Searching the World Wide Web

The Internet provides a variety of information sources. Be sure, however, to choose the sources you use wisely. There is as much bad information on the worldwide web as there is good. Use sound judgment and consider the following factors:

- What is the date of the information? Make sure it is not outdated.

- Is it coming from a reputable and well-known source? Information coming from a major hospital or university is generally more credible than coming from an unknown practitioner – particularly one whose interest is in selling a product.

- Be careful of information from cancer organizations unless they are well known.

- Usually information from libraries, government agencies and professional journals is trustworthy.

Always discuss any information you find on the Internet with your doctors or nurses before you try, join, or buy anything.

Books and Magazines

There are many publications issued by legitimate health care and caregiver organizations that you may find helpful as a source of information and/or support. As in evaluating Internet sources, consider the source. Who is publishing the information? Are they credible? Are they asking you for money for information?

Phone Support/Chat Rooms

This is an area that requires you to be very cautious. Phone and Internet chat rooms can be very dangerous. As a rule, do not seek or accept advice from chat rooms or telephone help lines. The exceptions to this rule are those from well-known and credible sources. Always be careful to protect your own identity and to discuss any information you receive with your health care professionals before you act on it.

Caution is the word when seeking information, but there are, however, many reliable sources from which you may seek information. Here are some of them.

American Brain Tumor Association – funds brain tumor research and provides information to patients, www.abta.org, 800-886-2282.

American Association of Retired People – offers useful information about advance directives, www.aarp.org, 800-424-3410.

American Cancer Society – provides written information about cancer, cancer research, and treatment options, www.cancer.org, 800-ACS-2345.

American Chronic Pain Association – has a network of 800 chapters that provide support for people dealing with chronic pain, www.theacpa.org, 916-632-0922.

American Geriatrics Society – provides information about making health care decisions; legal, ethical and financial issues, www.americangeriatrics.org, 212-308-1414.

American Red Cross – depending upon the community in which you live, may provide transportation for medical appointments, home-delivered meals, support groups, and friendly visitors, www.redcross.org.

American Pain Society – provides information about pain treatment centers in the U.S., www.ampainsoc.org, 847-375-4715.

Brain Tumor Society – provides resources for patients, survivors, families, friends, and professionals, www.tbts.org, 800-770-TBTS.

Brave Kids – resource for support services for children with life-threatening and terminal illnesses. www.bravekids.org, 415-561-2393.

Cancer Information Services – a network of regional offices sponsored by the National Cancer Institute. Provides information on cancer treatment, research and resources, http://rex.nci.nih.gov, 800-4-CANCER.

Cancer Survival Toolbox – a free set of cancer patient education audio tapes developed by a number of cancer organizations, 877-866-5748, www.cansearch.org.

Candlelighters Childhood Cancer Foundation – a not-for-profit organization that provides support groups for children, parents and caregivers. www.candle-lighters.org, 800-366-2223.

CaP CURE – identifies and supports prostate cancer research, www.capcure.org, 800-757-2873.

Caregiver.com – provides an online newsletter with caregiver tips, www.caregiver.com.

Partnership for Caring: America's Voices for the Dying – offers booklets on various end-of-life issues, including advance directives. You can also get your state's laws on medical decision making from this web site, www.choices.org, 800-989-9455.

Encore Plus – a program of the YWCA that provides women under treatment and recovering from breast cancer with a combined peer support group and exercise program, www.ywca.org.

Gilda's Club — provides meeting places, support and networking groups, lectures, workshops, and social events in a nonresidential, homelike setting, www.gildasclub.org, 1-888-GILDA-4-U.

Hospice Foundation of America – provides general information about hospice care, www.hospicefoundation.org, 800-854-3402.

International Myeloma Foundation – provides patient myeloma education and advocacy, www.myeloma.org, 800-452-2873.

Leukemia and Lymphoma Society of America – provides local support groups and limited financial assistance to people with leukemia, lymphoma, and multiple myeloma, www.leukemia.org, 800-955-4572.

MAMM – a magazine for women living with breast and reproductive cancers, www.MAMM.com, 212-243-2916.

National Cancer Institute – coordinates the national cancer program, which conducts and supports research, training, and other programs, www.cancer.gov, 800-4-CANCER.

National Coalition for Cancer Survivorship – works for quality cancer care for all by empowering survivors, www.cansearch.org, 888-NCCS-YES.

National Family Caregivers Association – advocates on behalf of caregivers through support, education, and awareness, www.nfcacares.org, 800-896-3650.

National Health Information Center – a health information referral service operated by the U.S. government, www.health.gov/nhic/, 800-336-4797.

National Hospice and Palliative Care Organization – helps find hospices and provides informational materials, www.nhpco.org, 800-658-8898.

National Institute on Aging – provides free materials on many topics, www.nih.gov/nia, 800-222-2225.

National Ovarian Cancer Coalition – raises awareness and promotes education about ovarian cancer, www.ovarian.org, 888-OVARIAN.

Needy Meds – provides free information about getting medications from pharmaceutical companies, www.needymeds.com.

Office of Minority Health Resource Center – part of the Department of Health and Human Services, offers guide to minority health resources, 800-444-6472, www.omhrc.gov/omhrc.

OncoLink – provides cancer-related information including reimbursement assistance and caregiver programs, www.oncolink.upenn.edu.

Oncology Nursing Society – organization of registered nurses that works with cancer patients and has a special section of their web site with patient information, www.ons.org, 412-921-7373.

Patient Advocate Foundation – provides education about managed care and financial issues for cancer patients, www.patientadvocate.org, 800-532-5274.

Pharmaceutical Research and Manufacturers of America – provides a directory of drug assistance programs, www.phrma.org, 202-835-3400.

Ronald McDonald House Charities – provides low cost lodging for families of children who are receiving treatment at nearby hospitals, www.rmhc.com, 630-623-7048.

Susan G. Komen Breast Cancer Foundation – provides information about breast cancer research and breast health and a toll-free volunteer "Helpline," www.breastcancerinfo.com, 800-IM-AWARE (800-462-9273).

Ulman Cancer Fund for Young Adults – provides support programs, education and resources, free of charge, to benefit young adults who are affected by cancer, www.ulmanfund.org, 888-393-FUND.

Us Too! International, Inc. – network of chapters that provide support for men with prostate cancer and their loved ones, www.ustoo.com, 800-808-7866.

Viatical Association of America – provides a list of companies that will buy your life insurance policy under certain conditions, www.viatical.org.

Well Spouse Foundation – an information and education organization for caregivers, www.wellspouse.org, 800-838-0879.

The Wellness Community — helps enhance health and well-being of cancer patients and their loved ones by providing a professional program of emotional support, education, and hope, www.wellness-community.org.

Y-ME National Breast Cancer Organization – provides support groups to individuals concerned about or diagnosed with breast cancer, including a men's support line for men whose partner has breast cancer, www.y-me.org, 800-221-2141.

GLOSSARY
OF COMMONLY USED TERMS RELATIVE TO CANCER

Benign
Not cancerous and does not spread from one part of the body to another

Biopsy
The surgical removal of tissue for examination to aid in diagnosis

Carcinogen
A substance that can cause cancer

Cancer
A group of diseases in which malignant (cancerous) cells grow out of control and spread to other parts of the body

Chemotherapy
The treatment of cancer with drugs

Clinical trial
A research project that a university, government entity, hospital, or other group may conduct to evaluate if a particular treatment process (such as chemotherapy, hormone therapy, radiation, or some combination of these) is effective

Hematologist
A doctor who specializes in blood and bone marrow problems

Immunotherapy/Hormone therapy
Treatment that uses certain parts of the body's immune system or hormones to fight cancer

Malignant
Cancerous cells that can spread to other parts of the body

Medicare
A government medical care program for older adults or patients who are disabled

Medicaid
Medical aid designed for those unable to afford regular medical service and financed by the state/federal governments

Metastasize
To spread to other parts of the body

Oncologist
A doctor who specializes in cancer treatment

Palliative care
Treatment geared toward supportive care rather than curative treatment

Radiation therapy
X-ray treatment that damages or kills cancerous cells

Risk factors
Anything increasing a person's chances of developing cancer; can be environmental or hereditary

Screening
Tests that are used to spot cancer early (even before symptoms occur)

Site
Body part in which cancer first develops (primary site)

Stage
The extent of the cancer in the body

Symptoms/side effects
Effects caused by drugs used for disease treatment such as pain, depression, anxiety, nausea, vomiting, etc.

Tumor
An abnormal overgrowth of cells that can be malignant (cancerous) or benign (non-cancerous)

ABOUT THE QUALITY OF LIFE FOUNDATION

The Quality of Life Foundation was started in 1993 in Indianapolis, IN, by William Dugan, Jr., M.D., and Sara Edgerton. These co-founders recognized the need for research efforts geared toward the quality of life of cancer patients to enable them to perform daily activities. The foundation's mission is to improve the quality of life of those affected by cancer, and their caregivers, through programs of research, education, and support.

About the Authors

Dale E. Theobald, Ph.D, M.D.
Dr. Theobald is a psychiatrist and Director of the Quality of Life Program for Community Cancer Care in Indianapolis, IN. He provides quality-of-life care for cancer patients and actively develops symptom control research protocols for Community Cancer Care's hospital partners.

Dr. Theobald has been an Assistant Clinical Professor of Psychiatry at the Indiana University School of Medicine in Indianapolis since 1987, and his research efforts have been published in several medical industry publications. He was recently appointed as Distinguished Fellow of the American Psychiatric Association and holds an endowed chair of Clinical Research in Oncology Symptom Management by the Methodist Health Foundation in Indianapolis. Dr. Theobald also previously co-owned and operated a private practice in psychiatry for twelve years.

William M. Dugan, Jr., M.D.
Dr. William Dugan, Jr. is the co-founder of the Quality of Life Foundation in Indianapolis, IN. He is also the co-founder and President of Community Cancer Care, a healthcare organization in Indiana that partners with more than 25 hospitals in rural and under-served areas to provide state-of-the-art cancer care and programming right in the local communities.

He is a medical oncologist/hematologist and has been in the oncology field for 39 years. He is on the teaching faculty and is an Assistant Clinical Professor of Medicine at the Indiana University School of Medicine in Indianapolis. He is also past national president of the Association of Community Cancer Centers and has been invited to testify before Congress in Washington D.C. about healthcare reform. Dr. Dugan has been named in the "Guide to Top Doctors," which identifies the top 15,000 doctors in the United States who are most highly recognized by their peers. His research efforts have been published in numerous medical industry publications.

Judy Burnett

Judy Burnett is the founder and director of Projects & Promotions — a division of Weiss Communications — an Indianapolis, IN, based public relations, event management, and marketing firm. She is a freelance writer as well, and contributes feature stories regularly to local, regional, and national publications. Judy's mother died several years ago after a short battle with lung cancer.

Abby A. Marmion

Abby Marmion owns and operates Chameleon Company, a marketing and public relations firm in Indianapolis, IN. Several of her clients are related to the medical industry. She is also a freelance writer. Abby has been touched by cancer through her family members.

Sara Edgerton

Sara Edgerton is co-founder of the Quality of Life Foundation along with Dr. Dugan. She is also co-founder and Chief Executive Officer of Community Cancer Care in Indianapolis, IN. She has been in the healthcare industry for more than 30 years and began her career with the Indiana Division of the American Cancer Society. She also owned and operated her own healthcare consulting company, specializing in marketing and business development for medical practices in various fields, including oncology, cardiology, and family practice. Sara has authored articles in several healthcare industry publications.

THE QUALITY OF LIFE FOUNDATION

The mission of the Quality of Life Foundation is to improve the quality of life of those affected by cancer, and their caregivers, through programs of research, education, and support. *The Strength to Fight Cancer - A Family Guide* is the first in what we hope will be a series of books to improve the quality of life of those affected by cancer.

We hope you found this book helpful. Copies are available free of charge upon request. If you would like to make a donation to further the work of the Quality of Life Foundation and to make possible the printing of additional books, your support would be welcomed.

Name _____

Address _____

City, State, Zip _____

Telephone _____

Please accept my donation to support the work of the Quality of Life Foundation

_____ $25 _____ $50 _____ $100 _____ Other

Please make checks payable to:

Quality of Life Foundation
115 West 19th Street
Indianapolis, IN 46202
317-924-4022

COMMENTS _____

_____

_____

_____

cut here

THE QUALITY OF LIFE FOUNDATION

The mission of the Quality of Life Foundation is to improve the quality of life of those affected by cancer, and their caregivers, through programs of research, education, and support. *The Strength to Fight Cancer - A Family Guide* is the first in what we hope will be a series of books to improve the quality of life of those affected by cancer.

We hope you found this book helpful. Copies are available free of charge upon request. If you would like to make a donation to further the work of the Quality of Life Foundation and to make possible the printing of additional books, your support would be welcomed.

Name _____

Address _____

City, State, Zip _____

Telephone _____

Please accept my donation to support the work of the Quality of Life Foundation

_____ $25 _____ $50 _____ $100 _____ Other

Please make checks payable to:

Quality of Life Foundation
115 West 19th Street
Indianapolis, IN 46202
317-924-4022

COMMENTS _____

_____

_____

_____

NOTES

NOTES

NOTES

NOTES

NOTES

NOTES

NOTES

NOTES